Old School Fitness Routines

Featuring Routines by:

EDWARD B. WARMAN

DANIEL L. DOWD

HARRY B. WEINBURGH

ADRIAN P. SCHMIDT

Research, Compilation, and Commentary by:

JEFF RAYMER

Cover Design by Dalia Liat Toth

Compilation and Commentary Copyright © 2014 Jeff Raymer

All rights reserved.

ISBN: 149960579X
ISBN-13: 978-1499605792

DEDICATION

To failure.
Without you, I never find success.

CONTENTS

1   Twenty-Minute Exercises   1

2   Exercises Scientifically Prescribed for Use of Dumb-Bells   9

3   Exercises for Developing Every Muscle in the Human Body   23

4   Health and Strength for Busy People   37

WARNING

It is advisable to consult a doctor prior to beginning any new exercise routine. Improperly performing any exercise, including the exercises listed in this book, can lead to physical injury. It is advisable to seek the advice of a qualified fitness professional, such as a personal athletic trainer, to verify proper form and dynamics when performing exercise routines such as those presented in this book.

1
TWENTY-MINUTE EXERCISES

"Vigorously yours" was the closing signature of Edward Barrett Warman (1847-1931.) Warman vigorously promoted physical activity and fitness for over 40 years in the late 1800's and early 1900's.

Warman's *Physical Training: The Care of the Body* was an 1885 book containing routines for physical exercise without apparatus, dumb-bell exercises, single Indian club exercises, and double Indian club exercises.

Warman's approach to physical exercise without apparatus evolved from calisthenics, to incorporate dynamic tension, as is evident in his 1918 *Tensing Exercises*, in which he recorded a thorough forty-minute exercise routine.

By 1921, at the age of 74, Warman had selected particular exercises from the tensing routine to create the twenty-minute exercise routine presented here. Of these exercises, Warman proclaims that by performing them every day of the year, "years will be added unto thy life and life unto thy years."

The text and photos are from Warman, Edward B. *Twenty-Minute Exercises*. New York: American Sports Publishing Company, 1921. Print.

Further descriptive text of the stationary running routine is from Warman, Edward B. *Physical Training Simplified: Complete, Thorough and Practical. The Whole Man Considered; Brain and Body. No Apparatus Required. Fully Adapted to the Needs of Both Sexes*. New York: American Sports Publishing Company, 1897. Print.

General Directions

Do not hold the breath during an exercise. Contract the muscles as though overcoming a natural resistance. When the muscle is brought to its greatest tension it should be held a moment and then relaxed.

After becoming familiar with the movements the time required to take all the exercises will not exceed twenty minutes.

Correct position of the body when standing and sitting, and correct carriage of the body when walking, together with full, deep breathing and right living, are essential to HEALTH.

The exercises, to be of the greatest benefit, should become a daily habit. The *minutes* faithfully spent *now* will reward you in *years* by and by.

Before Arising

Lie flat on the back. Stretch the entire body, tensing and relaxing the muscles of the neck, arms, back, chest, abdomen and legs. This increases heart action and causes arterial distention in the most natural and effective manner.

After Arising

Cleanse the teeth, rinse the mouth, gargle, drink one or two glasses of cold water, then take all the exercises in the order given; take them vigorously but not violently.

Follow the exercises with a suitable bath (preferably cold if there is sufficient vitality for reaction); at least such a bath as is more suited to the needs of the body than to the whims of the mind.

For Neck, Upper Chest and Back

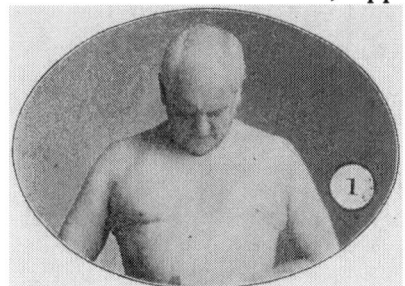 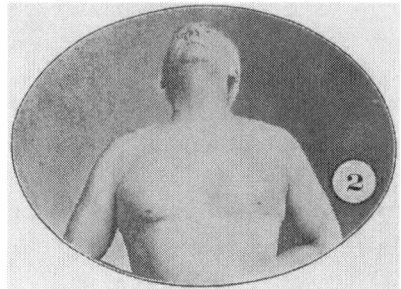

Body erect; head well poised. Move head forward and down (slowly), pressing chin to chest; then up, back and down. In both cases as far as possible *and then some.*

15 Times Each Way, Without Stopping

For Neck, Upper Chest and Back

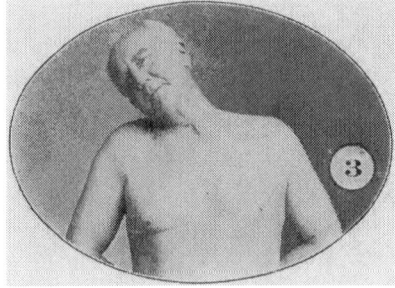 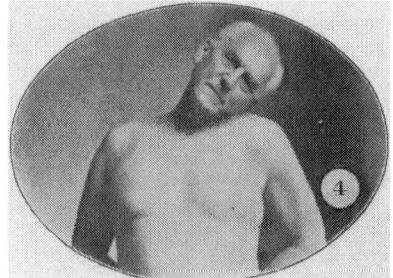

Body erect; head well poised. Move head toward right and left side, slowly, without turning the head. Try to touch ear to shoulder, without raising the shoulder or swaying the body.

10 Times Each Way, Without Stopping

For Neck, Upper Chest and Back

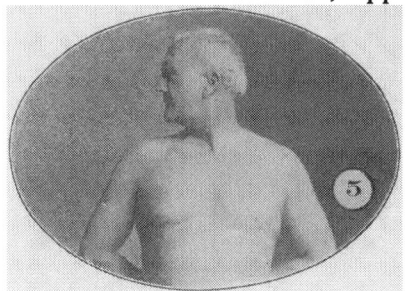 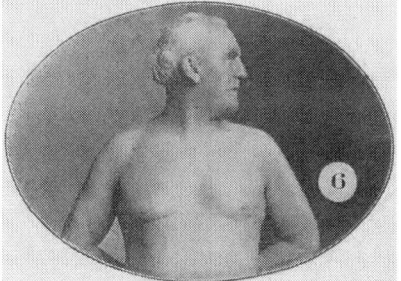

Body erect; head well poised. Turn head to right and left, very slowly, until chin is over shoulder. Do not tip the head forward or backward when turning. Do not turn the body.

5 Times Each Way, Without Stopping

For Calf and Forearm

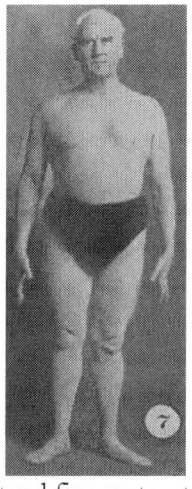 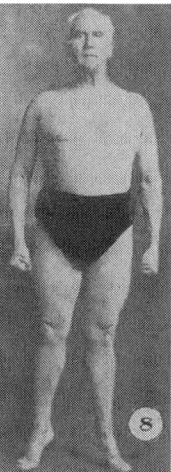

Body erect. Extend fingers to utmost limit with strong tension. Rise on toes, slowly, as high as possible, closing the hands with the strongest tension. Descend, slowly, to first position, again extending fingers to utmost limit.

50 Times

For the Upper Arms

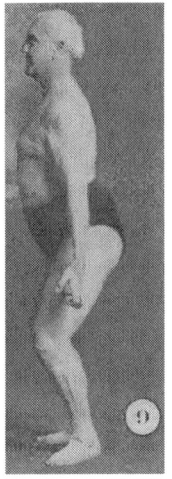 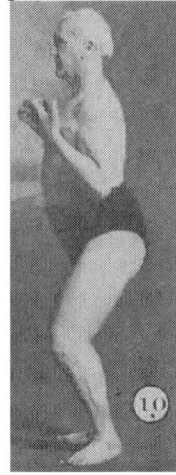

Body erect. Lower the body by bowing the legs. Tense the arms and half-closed hands. Retain leg position while slowly lifting a very heavy imaginary object with arms only. Contract the biceps to fullest extent; hold a moment, relax, tense the arms again, push down, very slowly, as against great resistance, thus contracting the triceps to the utmost. Retain leg position throughout.

7 Times

For the Thighs

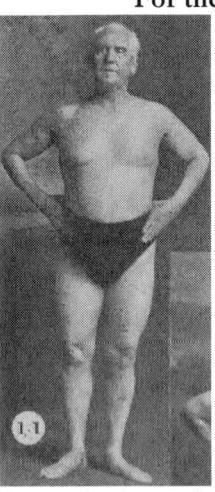 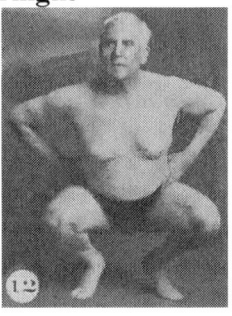

Body erect. Lower body to deep-knee bend and rise immediately to first position. In descending, allow the heels to rise from floor and close leg completely, lower thigh resting on upper calf.

25 Times

For the Thighs

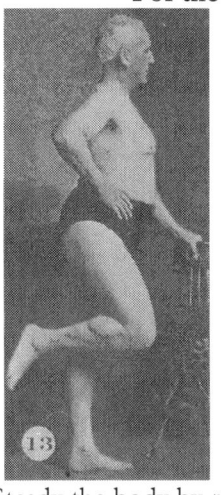 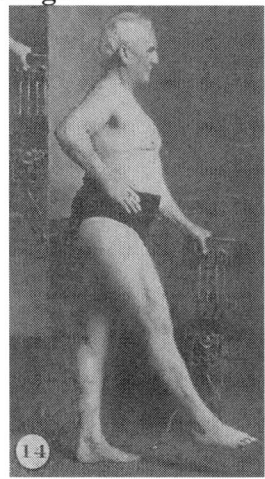

Body erect. Steady the body by resting the hand on back of chair while lifting the right foot and kicking vigorously 50 times.

Repeat the same with the left foot 50 times.

50 Times Each Foot

For Abdomen, Shoulders and Back

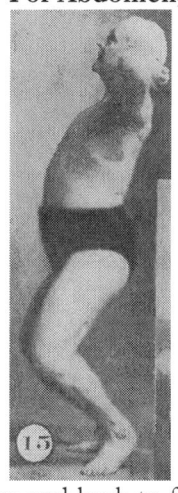 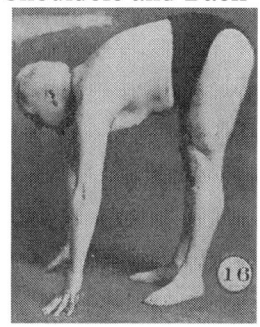

Swing arms up and back to first position, bending backward. *Be sure to bend the knees.*

Swing upward and forward, extending arms above, front and down, trying to touch the floor with the fingers, knuckles or palms. *Do not bend the knees.* Do not stop until movements are completed.

50 Times

For Abdomen, Shoulders and Hips

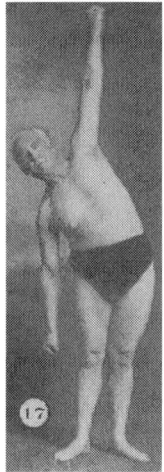 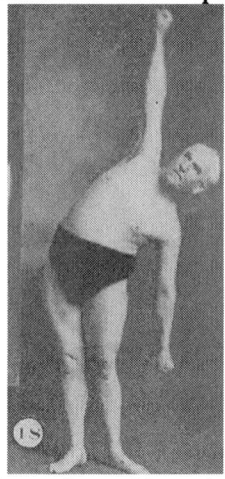

Swing left arm (strongly tensed) out from side and up to highest point; the right arm (strongly tensed) pulling down to lowest point.

Swing right arm up and left hand down in same manner, both arms strongly tensed.

25 Times

The Liver Squeezer

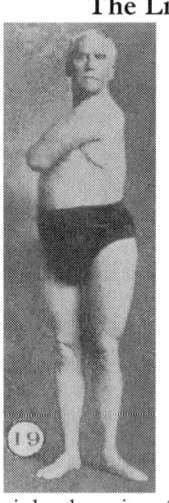 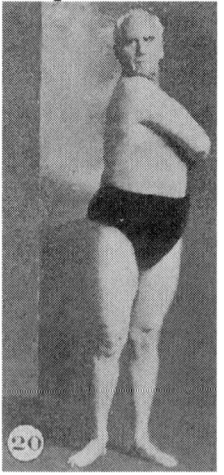

Twist body to right, keeping face to front, bringing left shoulder under chin, left arm across chest, right arm tense and extended close to body.

Reverse by twisting body to left, face kept front, bringing right shoulder under chin as you cross the chest with right arm; left arm tense and extended close to body. Strike across the chest vigorously, but not violently. Do not move the feet.

15 Times

For Chest, Shoulders and Back

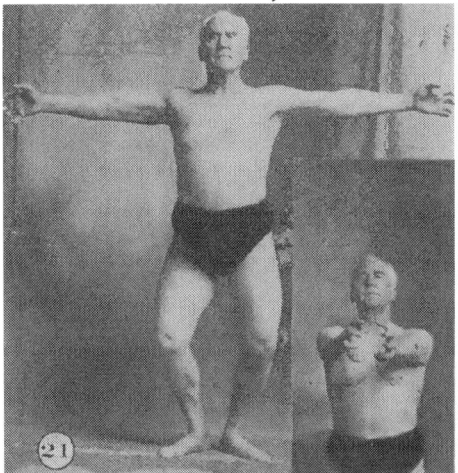 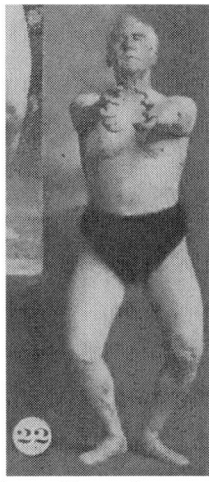

Body erect. Lower the body by bowing the legs. Extend arms at side on level with shoulders. Tense the arms and half-closed hands. Swing arms front and back, *without lowering*. Keep *strong tension* until completing the exercise. Do not sway the body.

25 Times

For Shoulders, Chest and Back

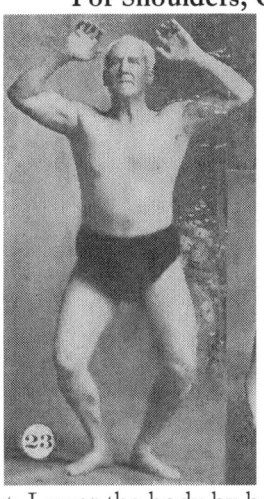 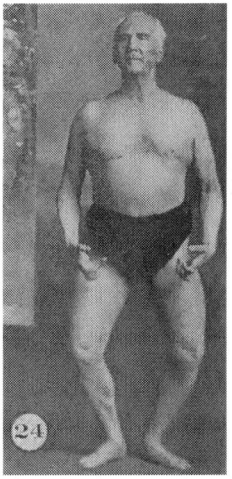

Body erect. Lower the body by bowing the legs. Raise the arms at side. Tense them to the utmost when starting them outward and downward *toward* but not quite *to* the body. Keep arms slightly bent at elbow. Relax the arms when raising them.

25 Times

For Legs, Lungs, Heart and Liver

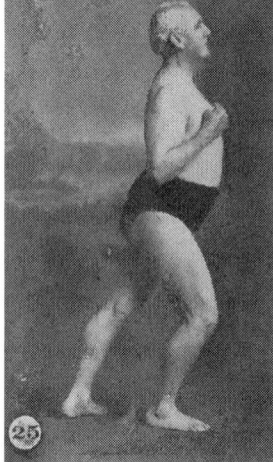

Stationary running. Hands to chest. Advance one foot. Incline body forward with weight on forward foot. Transfer the weight from foot to foot; as in actual running, except advancing. Keep mouth closed not only during, but after running until the breathing is normal. Run slowly and steadily. I take seven minutes for one thousand steps.

Begin with 100 Steps; Increase to 1,000

> Warman's 1897 *Physical Training Simplified* contains additional detail regarding the stationary running routine.

Incline the body forward as if starting to run, a race. Close the hands and place them on the chest to keep it active and to keep the arms from swaying. Close the mouth and *keep it closed.* Run, but do not move out of the position in which you are standing. Begin slowly, increase the speed, then more slowly again at the finish. Stand in the open, moving air, if possible, if not, by an open window.

Note: Count (mentally) each step as the foot touches the floor.

2
EXERCISES SCIENTIFICALLY PRESCRIBED FOR USE OF DUMB-BELLS

> *Prof. D. L. Dowd's System: How to Obtain an Even Development of all the Muscles of the Human Frame, Thereby Gaining Health and Strength; Something That is Within the Reach of Every Man, Woman and Child* was published in 1883 by the "Champion Heavy Weight Lifter of the World."
>
> In this slim eight page book, Professor Dowd presented his dumb-bell routine and stated, "You may think from the looks of this pamphlet that there can't be much worth in it, but I give you my word it is worth hundreds of dollars to anyone who is in the need of physical training, and any man, woman or child who hasn't got a good, robust, straight, healthy body, is sadly in need of it."
>
> By 1886, Professor Dowd had expanded his work to 300 pages in length, and included a comprehensive discussion of vocal exercise, abdominal breathing, facial exercise, skin care, posture, pulley exercises, and the dumb-bell routine in his *Physical Culture for Home and School: Scientific and Practical*. The line drawings included for the dumb-bell routine in this work had not been present in Dowd's prior text.
>
> A smaller book containing only the dumb-bell routine was published in 1888. Presented here is that version of text and line drawings from Dowd, D. L. *Exercises Scientifically Prescribed for Use of Dumb-Bells*. New York: Private Edition; Printed for the Author, 1888. Print.
>
> Additional information from the original work which followed the description of each exercise has been omitted here. That additional information featured a description of the muscle and its function.

Dumb-Bell Exercises

A great deal of benefit, physically, can be derived from the use of dumb-bells, but in order to gain it you must understand how to use them in an intelligent and scientific manner. Many people have resorted to the use of dumb-bells to better their physical condition; they have bought a pair of bells of a weight ranging from ten to a hundred pounds, and set to work with them without any special direction as to how they should be used to the best advantage. Indeed, I think the great majority of those that have indulged in the use of them have done themselves more harm than good, more especially those who have used heavy weights; and the rest have become tired because they did not know how to use them, thus losing their interest in the work. The performer should have understood that there is a special exercise for every set of muscles in the body, and just how to apply it.

In the following pages you will find special exercises for some of the prominent muscles of the body, arms, and legs. Many of them can be developed by the intelligent use of dumbbells.

One great drawback to the use of dumbbells is the monotony of the work; but if you will, you can do yourself considerable good by their use.

In using bells remember the following hints:

First: You must practice at least five times a week, but if you can practice once every twenty-four hours so much the better; the whole exercise will not last over forty-five minutes.

Second: You must work every muscle until you have tired it, and make it ache a little. From this light exercise the muscles will recover their strength very quickly. Always stand erect, with the head up and the chest projected.

For business people about 4 p.m. is generally thought the best time to exercise, for it is this time that the general depression from business is most keenly felt; hence the reason for livening up before the evening meal by a little exercise. If you cannot take this hour, then almost any time of day or evening will do.

Third: When performing with the dumb-bells, be sure not to swing the arms, I mean that swing that is given to them by a motion of the body, but raise and lower them by the power of the muscles, and not the swing.

Fourth: Make all the movements fairly quick and even; do not make any jerky movements. Bear in mind that you must not tire the muscles to the fullest extent until you have practiced for about two weeks.

Fifth: From five to eight pounds for each bell should be used. The strongest should not use more than eight pounds. Ladies should use from three to five pounds according to the strength.

Sixth: You must practice the exercises in the order in which they are here given, as they have been arranged to the best advantage.

> In his 1883 work, Dowd discussed the method of determining how to select an appropriate dumb-bell weight.

Stand erect, with arms hanging at the sides, palms turned in; now raise them with the backs turned up as high over the shoulder as you can lower them again to the sides; now whatever the weight may be that you can hold in your hands in this position, and raise about 20 or 25 times and have them thoroughly tire your shoulders and make them ache a little, is the exact weight you want for all your exercise. You will never need to change them for heavier ones, but as you grow stronger you will naturally raise them a greater number of times.

> In the accompanying images, the major muscle being worked in each exercise is denoted with a leader and the number 1 (and sometimes 2.)

Dumb-Bell Exercise No. 1
Lateral Portion of the Deltoid Muscle, on the Side of the Shoulder

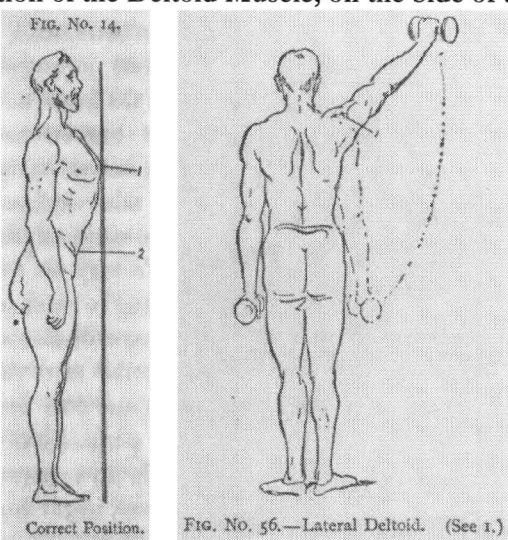

Correct Position. FIG. No. 56.—Lateral Deltoid. (See 1.)

Take a bell in each hand, with the palms turned toward the outside of the thigh, and maintaining the body erect, the feet together, the hips drawn back, the chest projected, the shoulders drawn back, the head erect, and the chin drawn in (see Fig. No. 14). Now, with the arms straight and stiff, raise them up both together (only one raised in figure) straight out and up from the sides of the body, and as high as you can (see Fig. No. 56). Repeat this movement until you tire the shoulder-muscles. Inhale strongly and deeply as the arms are ascending, and exhale forcibly as the arms are descending.

Take breath this way ten or a dozen times, and then fill the lungs comfortably full and hold the breath in while you make three or four movements, or as many as you can conveniently; then let it out, and repeat it until you feel that you have tired the lungs slightly.

> Figure 14 is missing from *Exercises Scientifically Prescribed for Use of Dumb-Bells*. As such, it is taken from Dowd, D. L. *Physical Culture for Home and School: Scientific and Practical.* New York: Private Edition; Printed for the Author, 1888. Print.

Dumb-Bell Exercise No. 2
Latissimus Dorsi, Muscle Covering the Side of the Back

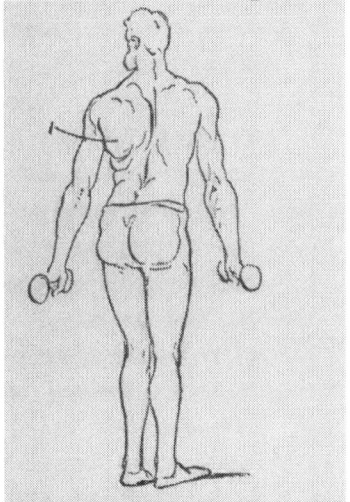

FIG. No. 57.—Latissimus Dorsi. (See 1.)

With a bell in each hand, stand with the body erect, the feet together, hips drawn back, the chest projected, the shoulders drawn back, the head erect, and the chin drawn in. Now, keeping the body as stiff as is possible, press the left arm downward as hard as you can, by drooping the shoulder, just as though you were pushing against some object on the floor that reached to your hand (see Fig. No. 57), then allow the arm and shoulder to assume their natural position again, and perform the same with the right arm; use the right and left alternately in this exercise until you tire the muscle named. (You may not at first get much satisfaction from this exercise, unless you happen to get it just right; but satisfaction will soon come, if you will persevere in the effort.

Dumb-Bell Exercise No. 3
Anterior Portion of the Deltoid Muscle on the Front of the Shoulder

Take a bell in each hand, with the palms turned to the front; stand with the body erect, feet together, hips drawn back, chest projected, shoulders drawn back, head erect, and chin drawn in. Now, with the arms straight and stiff, raise them up both together, straight out and up in front of the body as high as you can (see Fig. No. 58). Repeat this movement until you tire that portion of the deltoid mentioned. Inhale strongly and deeply as the arms are ascending, and exhale strongly as the arms are descending. Take the breath in this way ten or a dozen times, and then fill the lungs comfortably full, and hold the breath in while you make three or four movements, or as many as you can conveniently. Then let it out, and repeat the same until you feel that you have tired the lungs slightly.

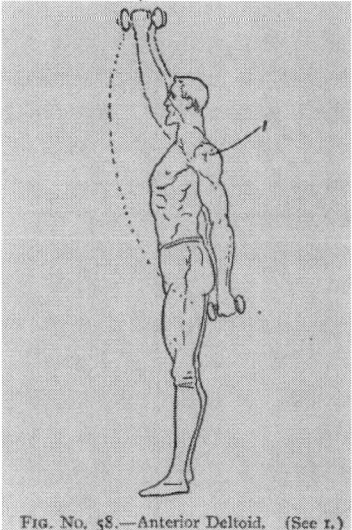

Fig. No. 58.—Anterior Deltoid. (See 1.)

Dumb-Bell Exercise No. 4
Muscles of the Forearm

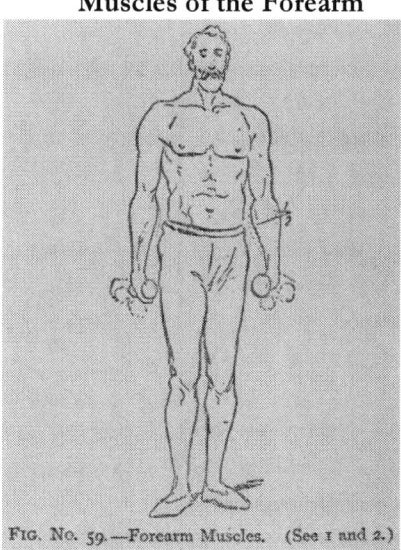

Fig. No. 59.—Forearm Muscles. (See 1 and 2.)

Take a bell in each hand, with the palms turned toward the outside of the thigh, with the body erect, feet together, hips drawn back, chest projected, shoulders drawn back, head erect, chin drawn in; now contract the inner portion of the forearm muscles, by bending the hand at the wrist inward and upward (see Fig. No. 59), then bend the hand at the wrist backward and upward. Repeat this movement with the hands at the same time; first turn them inward as strongly as you can, and then turn them backward as strongly as possible until you make the muscles of the forearm ache.

Dumb-Bell Exercise No. 5
Muscles on the Sides of the Abdomen, Obliquus Abdominis

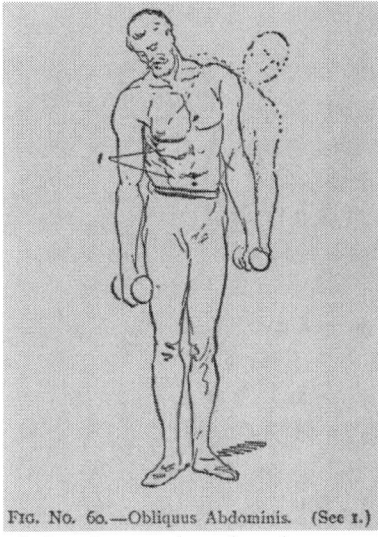

FIG. NO. 60.—Obliquus Abdominis. (See 1.)

Take a bell in each hand, arms hanging down at the sides. Stand erect, feet together, hips drawn back, chest projected, shoulders drawn back, head erect, chin drawn in. Now bend the body sideways, and a little forward; bending only at the hips sideways as far as possible, then rise, and bend over the other side in the same manner (see Fig. No. 60).

Take the breath in as the body is going from the right side to the left, and exhale as it is going to the right. Do so a few times, and then reverse the action of taking in the breath; after breathing this way a few times, take in quite a full breath, and hold it while you make as many movements as you can conveniently without feeling any strain. Then exhale, and repeat the exercise until you have tired the muscles. Should the lungs get tired before the muscles do, then stop the special breathing and continue the movement.

Dumb-Bell Exercise No. 6
Muscles on the Front of the Upper Arms, Biceps

With a bell in each hand, arms hanging down straight and palms turned to the front, stand with the body erect, feet together, hips drawn back, chest projected, shoulders drawn back, head erect, and chin drawn in. Now, keeping the elbows firmly at the sides, raise the bells to the shoulders by bending the arms at the elbows (see Fig. No. 61). Lower the bells to the sides again, and repeat the movement until you make the muscles ache; be sure and give them the full contraction, by allowing the arms to straighten fully, and then to move upward to the highest point possible each time.

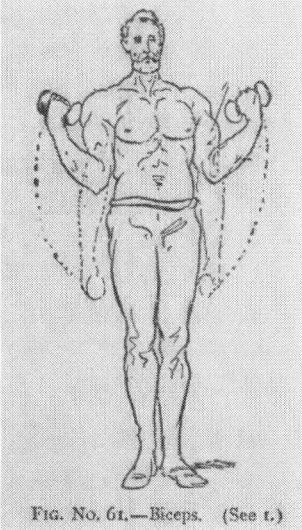

Fig. No. 61.—Biceps. (See t.)

Dumb-Bell Exercise No. 7
Loins of the Back, Erector Spinæ

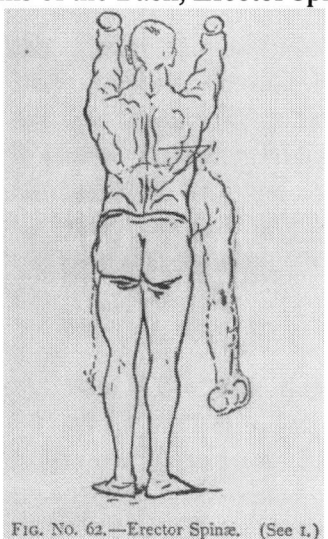

Fig. No. 62.—Erector Spinæ. (See t.)

With a bell in each hand, body erect, feet together, hips drawn back, chest projected, shoulders drawn back, head erect, and chin drawn in. Now, keeping the knees stiff, incline forward and downward (bending only at the hips), letting the bells come as near the floor as possible. Then, with the arms rigid and straightened out at full length in front of you, raise the body upward and bend a little backward (see Fig. No. 62). The arms should be held rigidly extended in front of the body all the time you are performing this movement; inhale deeply as the body moves forward and downward, and exhale forcibly as the body is moving upward and backward.

Dumb-Bell Exercise No. 8
Muscles on the Back of the Upper Arm, Lateral and Posterior Portions of the Triceps Muscles

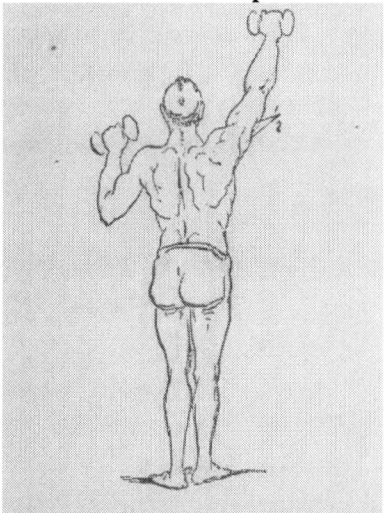

FIG. No. 63.—Triceps Muscles. (See 1 and 2.)

With a bell in each hand, raise the hands to the shoulders by bending the arms at the elbows. Stand with the feet together, body erect, hips drawn back, chest projected forward; shoulders drawn back, head erect, chin drawn in. Now elevate the bell in right hand straight above the head, extending the arm at full length (see Fig. No. 63); then draw the right arm back to the shoulder again, and while doing so extend the bell in left hand, straight above the head, thus exercising the left and right arm alternately. Continue this exercise until you have tired the muscles named.

Dumb-Bell Exercise No. 9
Muscles of the Breast, Pectoralis Major

Bell in each hand, body erect, feet together, hips drawn back, chest projected, shoulders drawn back, head erect, and chin drawn in.

Now, keeping the arms very rigid, move them across the body in front as far as you can, meanwhile keeping the elbows stiff and straight; see that the arms are kept close to the body, and allow them to cross each other (see Fig. No. 64); then move them back to place, and repeat the movement until you have tired the muscles named (the faithful practice of this exercise will bring about a very rapid and beneficial development).

Inhale the breath as the muscles are relaxing and the arms are moving from the front of the body to the sides, and exhale strongly as the arms are moving from the sides forward and across the body.

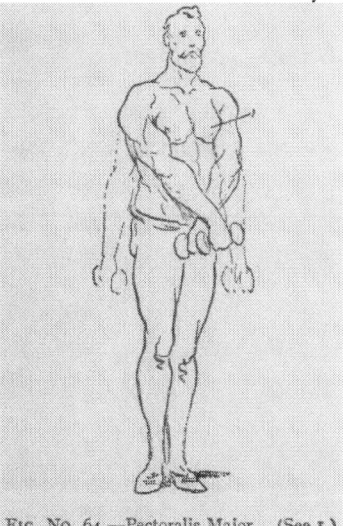

FIG. No. 64.—Pectoralis Major. (See 1.)

Dumb-Bell Exercise No. 10
Middle Portion of the Trapezius Muscles of the Back

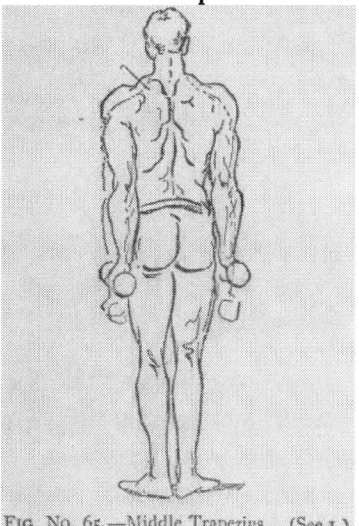

FIG. No. 65.—Middle Trapezius. (See 1.)

Bell in each hand, the arms straight at the sides of the body, body erect, feet together, hips drawn back, chest projected, shoulders drawn back, head erect, and chin drawn in. Now for the movement. Make an effort to raise the shoulders upward (keeping the arms perfectly straight; see Fig. 65) as high as you can, making a movement called shrugging of the shoulders. Repeat this movement rapidly until you have tired the muscles named, which will not take many seconds if you contract the muscles fully each time.

Dumb-Bell Exercise No. 11
Posterior Portion of the Triceps Muscles

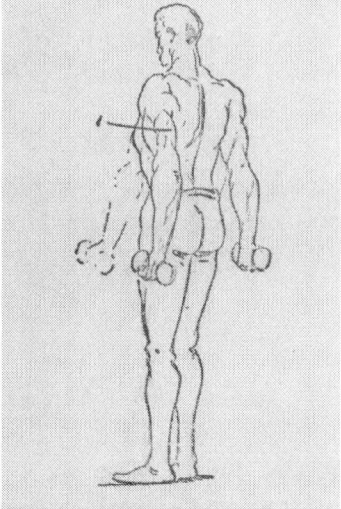

FIG. No. 66.—Posterior Triceps. (See ?.)

Bell in hand, body erect, feet together, hips drawn back, chest projected, shoulders drawn back, head erect, and chin drawn in. Hold the arms straight at the sides, with the palms turned to the front; now raise the arms (both together) backward as high as possible, and at the same time twist them *outward* as much as possible. This twisting is the most important part of this movement, so you must be sure and get it right. Twist the arms outward and backward as hard as you can, so that the backs of the hands will approach each other (see Fig. No. 66). Inhale deeply as the arms are moving backward, and exhale strongly as the arms are coming forward again; repeat until you tire the muscles.

Dumb-Bell Exercise No. 12
Posterior Portion of the Deltoid Muscles on the Back of the Shoulder

Bell in each hand, body erect, feet together, hips drawn back, chest projected, shoulders drawn back, head erect, and chin drawn in.

Turn the palm of the hand in toward the outside of the thigh, pitch the body a little forward, bending at the hips (so that your arm may rise higher); now move the right arm straight backward and upward, as high as you can without twisting the arm in any way (see Fig. No. 67); then lower to its place and do the same with the left arm, and make the movement with the right and left arm alternately, until you tire the muscle.

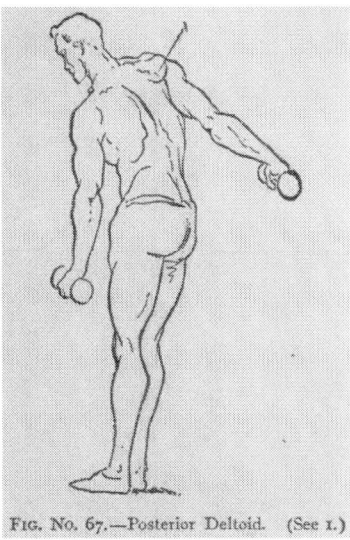

FIG. No. 67.—Posterior Deltoid.   (See I.)

Dumb-Bell Exercise No. 13
Muscles on Front of the Thighs, Quadriceps Extensor

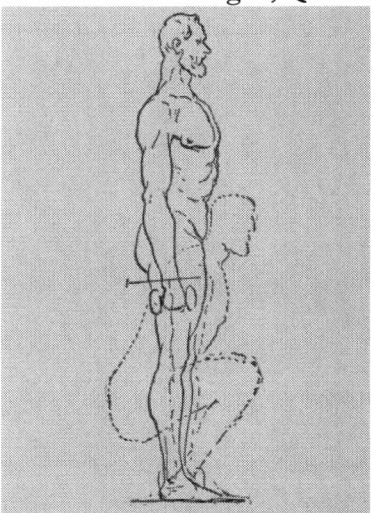

FIG. No. 68.—Quadriceps Extensor.   (See I.)

Bell in each hand, body erect, feet together. hips drawn back, chest projected, shoulders drawn back, head erect, and chin drawn in; now drop the body as near the floor as you can, bending at the hips and knees (see Fig. No. 68); then rise and repeat the movement, until you tire the muscles of the thighs.

Inhale as the body is lowering, and exhale strongly as the body is rising. This movement is what one could correctly term squatting.

Dumb-Bell Exercise No. 14
Muscles of the Calf, Gastrocnemius and Soleus

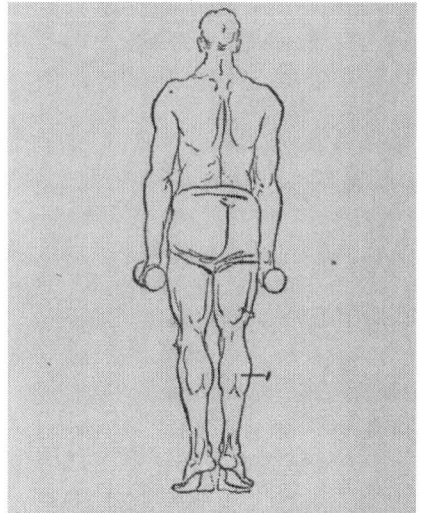

FIG. No. 69.—Gastrocnemius and Soleus. (See 1.)

Bell in each hand, body erect, feet together, hips drawn back, chest projected, shoulders drawn back, head erect, and chin drawn in. Hold this position and rise as high as possible on your toes (see Fig. No. 69). Repeat this movement until you have tired the muscles. Bear in mind that you must rise as high as possible each time, if you would gain the best results.

Dumb-Bell Exercise No. 15
Muscles on the Back of the Thighs, Biceps

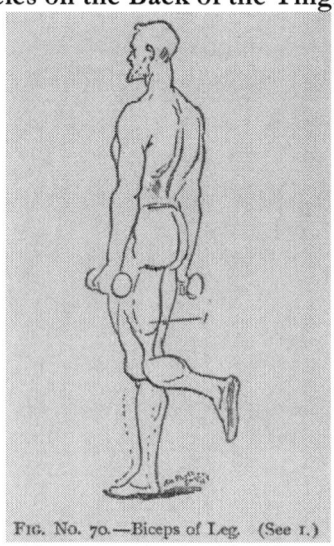

FIG. No. 70.—Biceps of Leg. (See 1.)

No bells this time, if you are tired of holding them; if not, hold them to steady yourself with.

Body erect, hips drawn back, chest projected, shoulders drawn back, head erect, and chin drawn in. Now raise the left leg upward from behind (bending at the knee) as high as you can; but do not let the left knee swing forward from the right, but hold it firmly against it (see Fig. No. 70). Lower to place again, and repeat the movement until you tire the muscle; then change to the right leg and tire that one. Be sure and rise as high as possible each time, and lower full length.

Dumb-Bell Exercise No. 16
Muscles on Front of Lower Leg, Tibialis Anticus

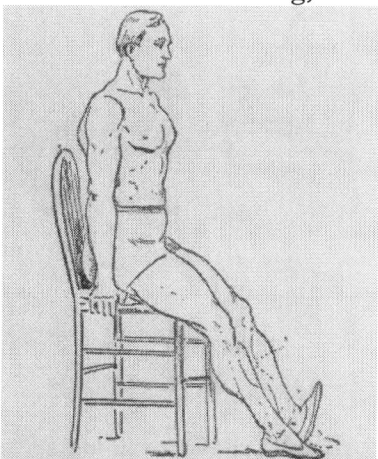

FIG. No. 71.—Tibialis Anticus. (See I.)

No bells. Sit in a chair or on a bench, and stretch your legs nearly at full length in front of you, with the heels pressed firmly on the floor; now move the toes toward the body as hard as you can, bending the foot at the ankle joint (see Fig. No. 71); then press them back again firmly, both feet together, and give the muscles the full contraction each time. Repeat the movement until you have tired the muscles mentioned.

Dumb-Bell Exercise No. 17
Muscles on Front of the Abdomen, Rectus Abdominis

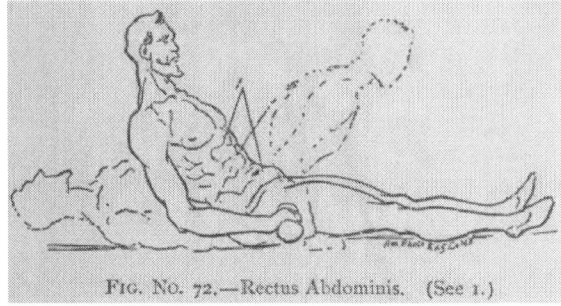

FIG. No. 72.—Rectus Abdominis. (See 1.)

Lie out at full length on a sofa, a bench, or on the floor; place your arms at the side or across your breast, as you choose; now raise the body from the prone to a sitting position (see Fig. No. 72); then lower it again. Repeat this movement until you feel that you have tired the muscles of the abdomen.

If this should prove to be too severe an exercise for you, then only lower the body part way down, until you gain more strength, if your legs seem to rise when you attempt to raise the body, then put some weight on them to keep them down.

3
EXERCISES FOR DEVELOPING EVERY MUSCLE IN THE HUMAN BODY

According to the title page of his book *Perfect Health: An Exhaustive Treatise on Natural Laws That Make and Maintain Perfect Health and Perfect Human Development; Written from Experience, Not Theory*, Harry Bennett Weinburgh was awarded the title of "Best Developed Man in America" in January 1902. In this book, Weinburgh states that "If all exercises here shown are practiced daily for a reasonable period of time each day, they will bring into active use and develop every muscle in the human body."

Weinburgh states that "Each movement should be taken from five to ten times, or until signs of fatigue are felt. Then change to another movement observing the same rule. The number of times a movement is taken can be increased each day until it can be executed twenty to twenty-five times without tiring."

The following photos and text are from Weinburgh, Harry Bennett. *Perfect Health: An Exhaustive Treatise on Natural Laws That Make and Maintain Perfect Health and Perfect Human Development; Written from Experience, Not Theory*. New York: Peter Eckler, 1903. Print.

In the original work, the exercise routine was dispersed throughout the book. The photos and descriptions were each separated by several pages of text in-between containing information about diet, medicine, sleep, and many other topics which are beyond the scope of this compilation. By bringing the routine together in one location, the text from the original work has been edited to omit references to figure numbers. It is the opinion of the compiler that since the figures are now aligned right beside each other, those frequent references to figure numbers are not necessary.

Exercise No. 1

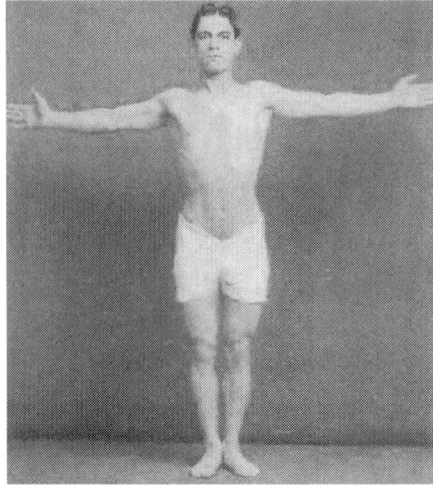

The arms should be extended as shown in figure; holding the shoulders high and pressed to the rear. This simple exercise taken every morning and the arms pressed from position to the rear as far as possible and back, alternately for a few minutes will in a short time give an erect and graceful carriage.

Exercise No. 2

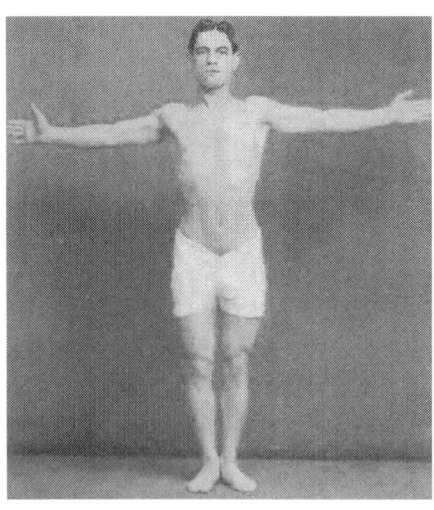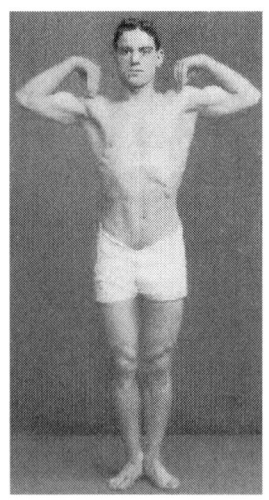

Tense the muscles and slowly press the hands to the top of the shoulders and return to position.

This movement should be taken as if lifting up and pushing down a heavy weight.

Inhale deeply as the hands are raised; exhale as they are lowered.

Exercise No. 3

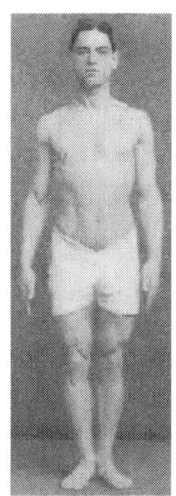 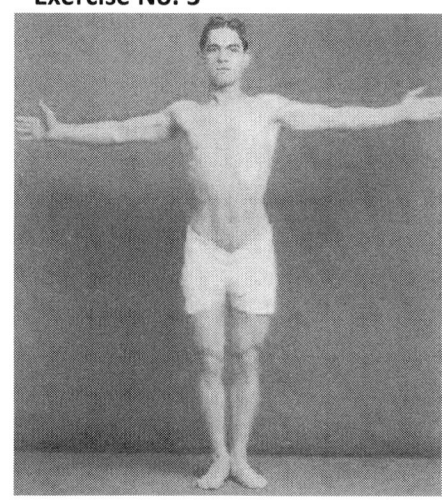

From this position press the arms slowly up to level with shoulders, tensing the muscles and stretching the arms to their utmost limit as if lifting and pushing down a weight.

Inhale with the ascending and exhale with the descending motion.

Exercise No. 4

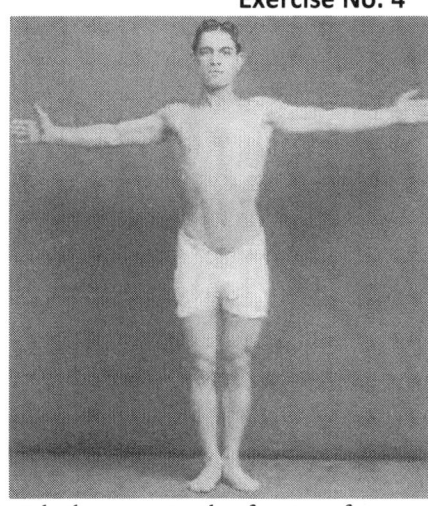 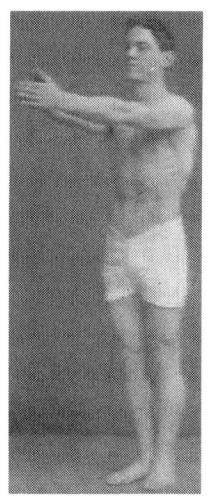

Outstretch the arms to the front as far as possible, tensing and pressing them to the rear, inhaling as the arms are forced backward and exhaling as they are brought forward.

This exercise can also be taken with a rapid motion, inhaling and exhaling with every two or three movements.

Exercise No. 5

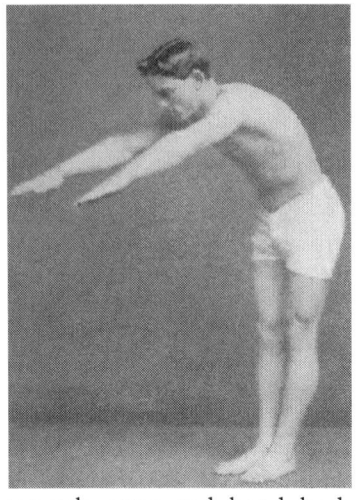 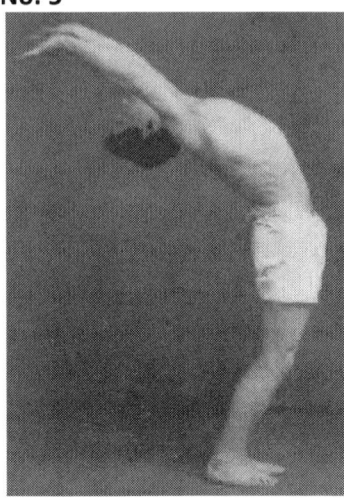

Outstretch arms and bend body from waist line forward as far as possible. Then bend backward.

This exercise should be taken slowly, inhaling with the backward and exhaling with the forward movement. It can also be taken rapidly inhaling and exhaling with each complete movement.

The daily practice of this exercise will lend to the body much grace and give it the suppleness necessary to accomplish this movement with ease.

Exercise No. 6

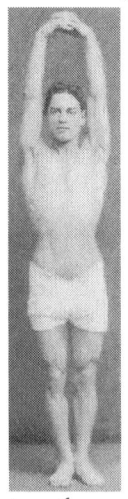 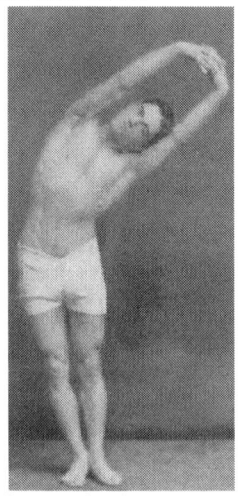

Keep the heels together and stretch the arms to their utmost height, clasping the fingers and holding the arms and body rigid; then bend from side to side. To derive most benefit from this movement, deep breathing should be practiced; inhaling as the body moves toward the right, and exhaling when bending to the left.

Care should be taken to keep the head resting on the lower arm with each movement.

Exercise No. 7

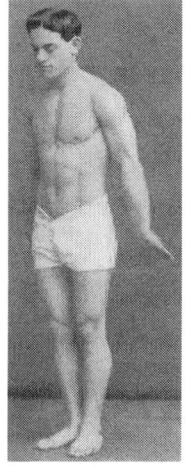
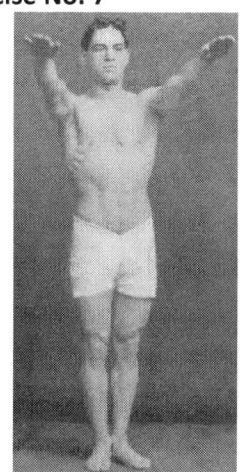

This gives the first position of an exercise I call "rolling the shoulders," which consists in describing a circle or wheel, making a hub of the shoulders and a rim of the hands.

Stretch the arms down to their full tension, bringing them forward. From this position elevate the arms close to the head, pressing them backward as far as possible in a circular motion to the beginning.

Inhale while making the upward and exhale while making the downward half of the circle.

Exercise No. 8

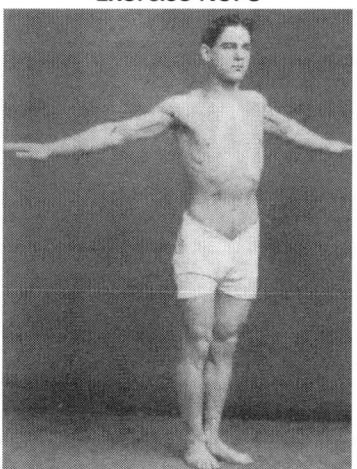

This is what I have named the "hoop" exercise.

It is taken with arms extended as shown in figure, and rolled with a quick motion, as if the wrists were encircled by a hoop.

The chest should be well extended and the rolling motion far to the rear.

Exercise No. 9

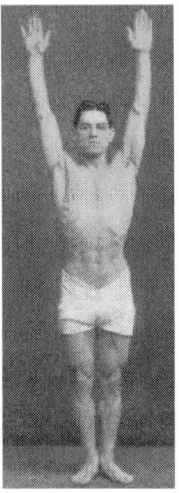
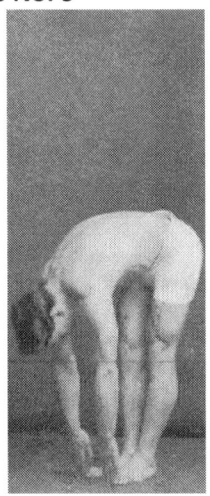

Stretch the body to its utmost height, bending slowly and reaching forward as far as possible without bending the knees, endeavoring to touch the floor in front of feet.

The position assumed in this movement is especially advantageous for deep breathing.

Inhale while ascending and exhale while descending.

Exercise No. 10

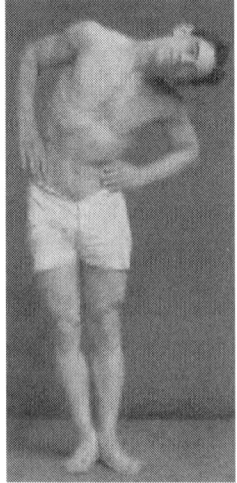

This illustrates an exercise especially recommended for strengthening the muscles of the neck and sides. It should be taken by moving the body at the waist line from side to side, inhaling from left to right and exhaling from right to left.

Exercise No. 11

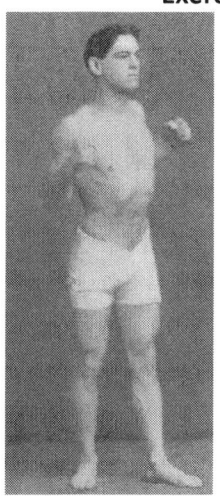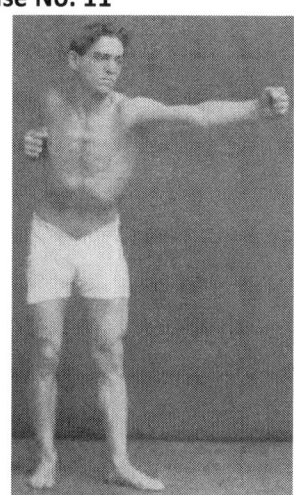

This shows a very valuable and vigorous exercise. Clinch the fists bringing them up at the sides with the shoulders pressed well towards the rear. Left foot forward.

Flex the muscles of the entire body; then strike out with the left hand at an imaginary object with all the force possible, so as to turn the body from the waist line.

The left hand should be brought back to position before striking with the right.

A second or two should intervene between strokes, and they should be alternated until signs of fatigue appear.

Exercise No. 12

From an erect position with hands on hips, bend the body only from the waist line, as far back as possible; then bend forward, keeping the knees rigid.

[This exercise] affords a splendid position for deep or diaphragmatic breathing.

Inhale while bending backward and exhale as the body is brought forward.

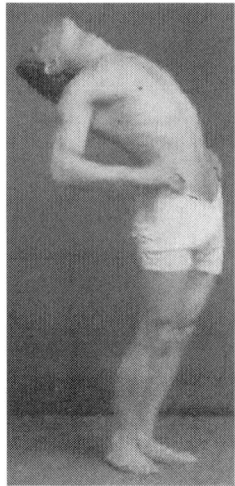 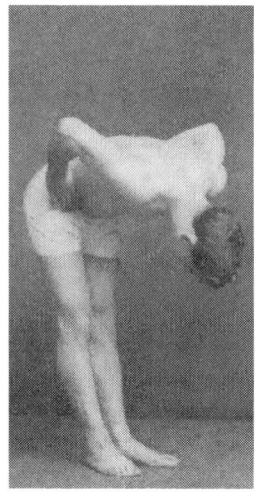

Exercise No. 13

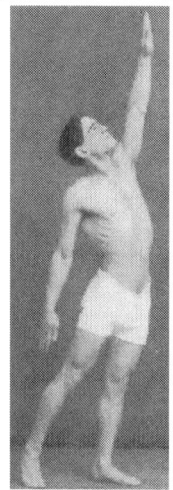

This illustrates one of my original stretching exercises.

But few people, even instructors, realize the great value of stretching or elongating the muscles and the body entire.

Inhale while slowly raising the left arm, retain the air for a few seconds, and stretch as if endeavoring to reach the ceiling with one hand and the floor with the other.

These movements can be alternated from six to a dozen times with great benefit, or until signs of fatigue are felt.

Exercise No. 14

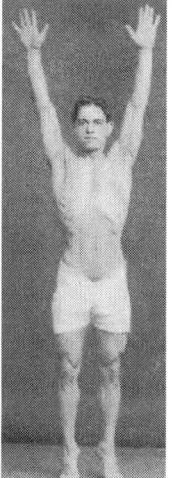

This movement I regard as one of the best of my stretching or growing exercises.

Extend the hands upward as shown in figure, at the same time inhaling a deep breath and rising upon the toes. Retain the air in the lungs for a few seconds, walking upon the toes and swaying from side to side, stretching the entire frame to its utmost.

I sincerely believe that it is to these stretching exercises that I owe several inches of my height.

Exercise No. 15

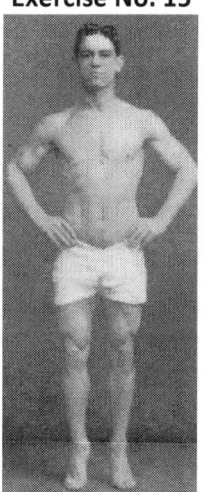

This exercise is especially recommended for the lower limbs.

The body should be elevated slowly to the position shown in figure and lowered in the same way. The exercise should be finished however with a few snappy movements.

The daily practice of this exercise will give to the carriage that lithesome and springy step so much admired and so much desired.

Exercise No. 16

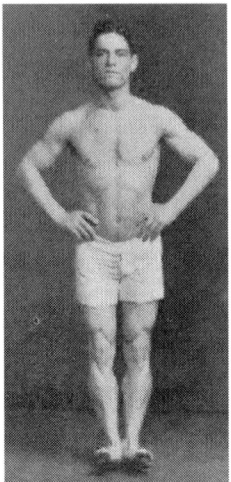

This exercise consists entirely in raising the toes as high as possible and lowering them to the floor while resting upon the heels. The body should be held erect and rigid while going through this movement.

This exercise, like [the previous exercise], is very beneficial for the front muscles of the lower limbs.

Exercise No. 17

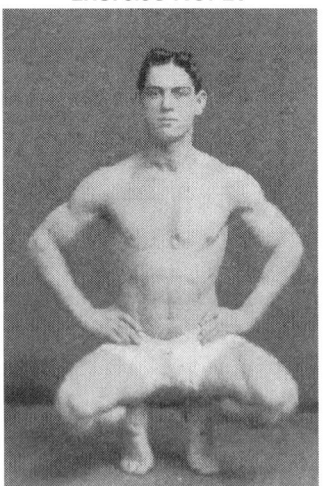

From the position shown in figure, slowly elevate the body to an erect posture and return to position. When rising, rest the full weight of the body on the toes.

This is one of the best movements known for strengthening all the muscles of the thighs and lower limbs, and is especially beneficial in Locomotor Ataxia.

Inhale while rising and exhale while descending.

Exercise No. 18

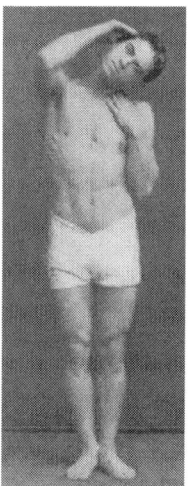

This illustrates an exercise for the neck.

Place the right hand on the side of the head; the left hand on the neck.

Force the head to the left as far as possible with the right hand; resisting this force with all the power in the neck muscles, alternate by changing the position of the hands. Repeat this movement about a dozen times toward each side.

Exercise No. 19

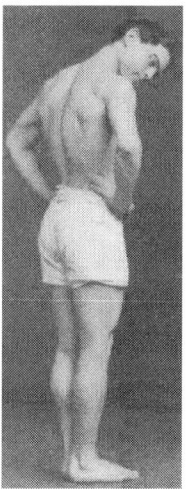

This is another Neck exercise and differs from [the previous exercise] in that it brings into action all the muscles of the neck without the use of the hands.

Place the chin on top of the left shoulder and move it slowly to the right with a downward circle almost touching the chest until it comes vertically over the right shoulder; resisting the movement with all the power possible.

This movement should be alternated from side to side from six to a dozen times.

Exercise No. 20

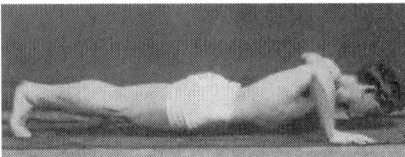 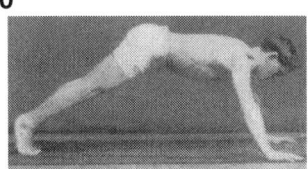

I would rather miss my dinner than miss this exercise. I regard it as one of the best movements for the entire frame, that is practiced in Physical Culture. Assume position as shown in this figure and elevate the body to the full limit of the arms, and return bending only at the waist line, as shown. In executing this movement raise the body slowly, elevating the hips as shown in this figure, and pushing backward without moving the feet; inhaling as the body is lowered and exhaling as it is raised.

The benefits from this exercise are largely increased by proper breathing, which is most always neglected in movements where the abdominal muscles are tensed or brought into active use.

Exercise No. 21

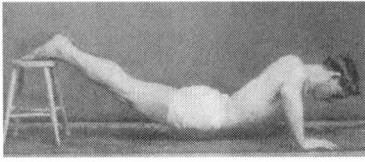 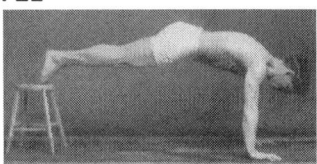

This figure illustrates an exercise similar to that shown in [the previous exercise], with the addition of a chair, which makes it more difficult. It should not be practiced until the [previous exercise] can be accomplished with some degree of ease.

The body should be raised to position shown. From this position lower the body to the posture shown in [the next figure], which completes the movement.

Inhale as the body is lowered and exhale as it is raised.

In all probability this exercise brings into use more muscles of the body at the same time than any one known to athletics.

It is especially good for weakened backs, spine and in cases of lumbago.

Exercise No. 22

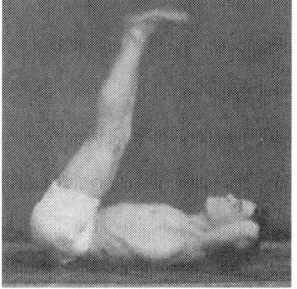

Begin this movement by lying at full length, elevating the feet to position shown in figure without bending the knees.

Inhale while lowering and exhale while elevating the feet.

A tendency to hold the breath is usually felt while practicing this exercise. This should be carefully avoided, for in order to get the full benefit from any exercise plenty of pure air should be taken into the lungs to purify the increased amount of blood that is forced there by the effort.

Exercise No. 23

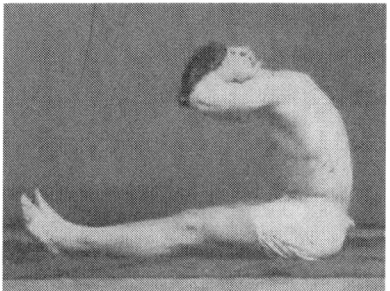

This movement is in effect much the same as [the previous exercise] with the addition of bringing into active use the muscles of the back and neck. If too much difficulty is experienced in raising the body with the hands clasped behind the neck they can be held by the sides.

Inhale as the body is lowered and exhale as it is raised.

Exercise No. 24

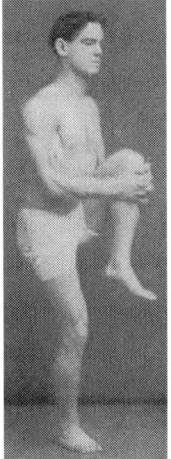

This movement I call "Abdominal Massage." It consists in pressing first one knee and then the other as far as possible towards the chest.

Inhale deeply every two or three movements according to lung capacity.

This movement is especially recommended for Indigestion and Constipation. It should be practiced for five or ten minutes morning and evening of each day.

Exercise No. 25

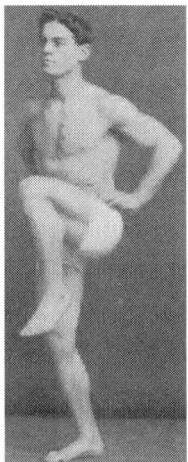

This movement I have named "Intestinal Exercise." It consists in bringing the knee with a quick motion towards the chest, lifting first one knee and then the other, with about the speed of a rapid walk.

The movement shown in this and also [the previous exercise] serve an especial purpose for the Intestinal machinery, because they give a movement that is never practiced in ordinary vocations.

4
HEALTH AND STRENGTH FOR BUSY PEOPLE

> Adrian Peter Schmidt says that his exercises "can safely be practiced by persons of middle age or beyond" and that his aim was to "present a practical manual for continuous use." Regarding the excellent drawings, Schmidt "spent considerable time and care upon the pen and ink drawings illustrating his instructions."
>
> Schmidt's book includes an endorsement by fourteen individuals attesting to the effectiveness of Schmidt's program. Among these is Clarence H. Mackay (1874-1938), of whom the United States National Aeronautic Association awards a yearly award in honor of. Other endorsers include artist Gustave Baumann (1881-1971) and E. W. Coggeshall, who wrote *The Assassination of Lincoln* and whose relative William Turner Coggeshall was a Lincoln bodyguard prior to the establishment of the Secret Service Division.
>
> Text and line drawings are from Schmidt, Adrian Peter. *Illustrated Hints for Health and Strength for Busy People*. New York: Adrian Peter Schmidt, 1901. Print.

My purpose is a very practical one; to suggest a simple plan for exercise in the morning, which will take only ten or fifteen minutes, but whose practical and beneficial results have been demonstrated in my experience as an advisor and instructor in physical culture.

The exercises do not require any apparatus and can be taken in a room large enough for you to turn around in with outstretched arms. Of course good ventilation is essential.

If you practice these exercises intelligently and persistently they will put you in a condition to go through your daily work with ease and pleasure.

To Stimulate Energy
Plate I

Here is a simple and rather ingenious plan to stimulate energy in a mild way on mornings when you do not feel inclined to exert your strength.

Take in each hand a corner of an ordinary sheet of newspaper (any kind of soft paper will do) and crumple it up until the four corners are brought into the palms of your hands, forming paper balls. Avoid assisting in the process by pressing the hands against the body. The result is surprising. Every muscle will be brought into sympathy with the muscles of the forearm in the effort to secure the last corner (to completely hide the sheets in your hands.) Your nervous force and blood circulation are thus pleasantly stimulated.

Practice this from one to two minutes, beginning slowly and gradually increasing in speed.

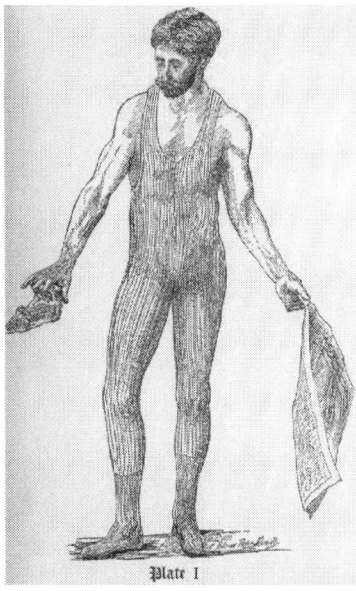

Plate I

For a Powerful Grip
Plate II

Remark: Using these paper balls in the same manner as a grip-machine, by grasping them as tightly as you can and then releasing the grip without opening the fingers entirely, repeating this about seventy-five times a minute, will insure a powerful grip. Simple as this paper grip-machine seems, it is superior in many ways to any manufactured device.

The writer has carried one in his coat pocket in cold weather to keep his hands warm by exercise and has repeatedly illustrated the strength of his fingers by tearing a corner off a full deck of cards, lifting with one finger a good-sized man by the belt, etc., feats that anyone can perform after persistent exercise.

This exercise does not make the hands callous nor enlarge or deform the joints. It massages the flesh covering the inside of the hands, including the thumb, and gives them beautiful outlines.

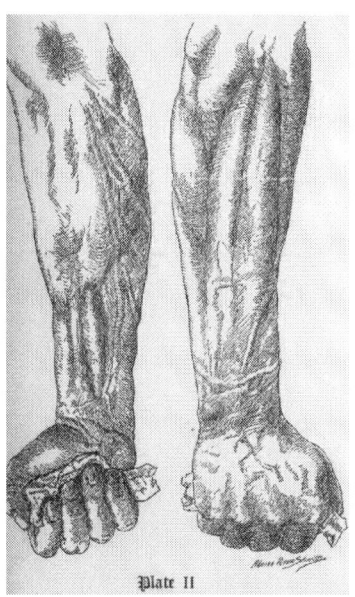

Plate II

For Supple, Strong Shoulders
Plate III

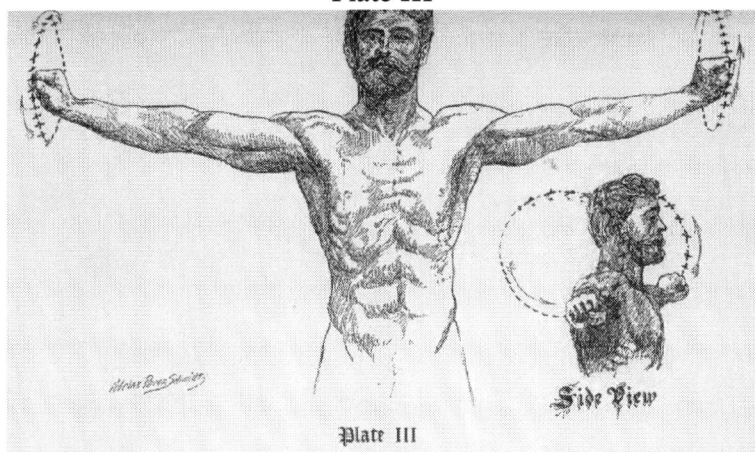

Side View

Plate III

Very effective exercise for the muscles of the neck, the upper trapezius muscles that cover most of the upper part of the back and deltoids or shoulder muscles.

Stand erect in a comfortable, natural position, bringing the outstretched arms sideways, with fists clinched, knuckles upward, elbows straight on a horizontal line with the shoulders. Compare your position in a mirror with illustration. (You can use paper balls for the convenience of having something to steady your fingers.)

Rotate arms, making fists travel in circles of about seven to ten inches in diameter, spending most of the energy on half circle marked with X on the dotted line.

For Supple, Strong Shoulders
Plate IV

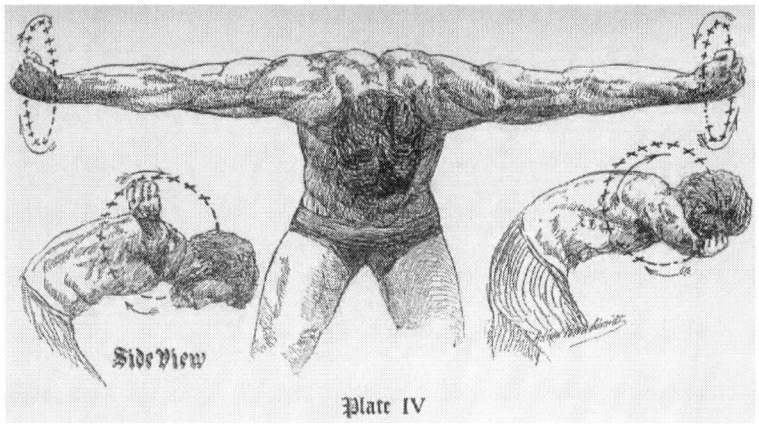

Arms the same as in Plate III, trunk inclined forward, knuckles downward. For convenience bring one leg forward, bending the knee as much as is comfortable. Reverse the rotation of your arms.

This exercise develops that part of the shoulder muscles, the absence of which your tailor supplies by padding your coat.

Begin the rotations slowly, laying stress on reaching as far sideways as possible, then gradually increase the speed. Continue the rotations for one minute in each position (III and IV) from forty to one hundred times, according to your strength. After this exercise the shoulders will require a rest.

For Strong, Shapely Ankles
Plate V

To stimulate the circulation in the lower extremities and develop the strength of their muscles.

Standing erect and without bending at the hips, raise heels and toes alternately from thirty to sixty times according to your strength and the time at your disposal. One minute will be sufficient.

Illustrations A, B, C and D show the various feet positions in which this exercise may be taken so as to bring into play the different calf muscles. It is advisable to take from eight to fifteen exercises in each position.

This exercise should be taken barefooted or in stockings on a soft rug. Raise as high as you can, avoiding dropping the heels suddenly.

If you have difficulty in keeping your balance, steady yourself by holding on to the back of a chair or to a door-knob.

Remark: Avoid going to extremes at first, as the calf muscles are liable to become painfully sore the next day.

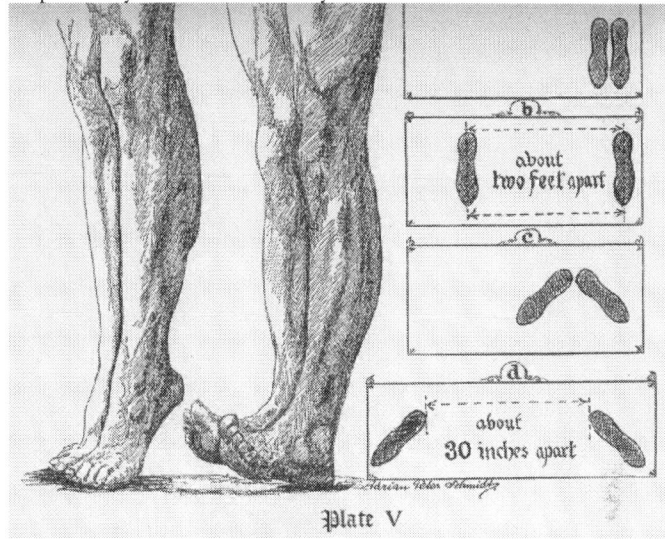

To Produce Good Circulation
Plate VI

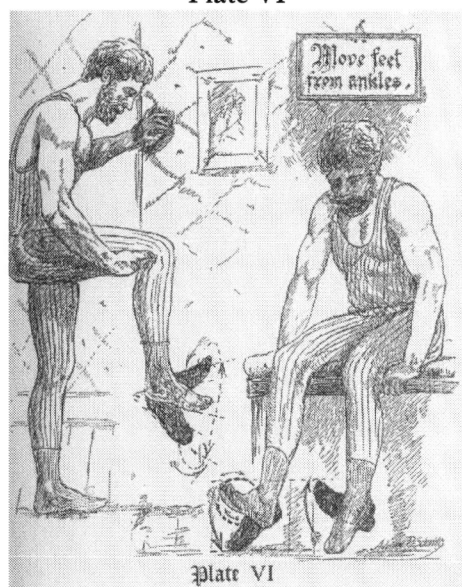

After previous exercise with the weight of your body alternately on the heels and toes, the accumulation of venous blood gives rise to a tired sensation in the leg muscles. To remove this temporary congestion immediately, lift the right foot off the floor, bending the knee, supporting the weight of the limb as shown in illustration IV. Move feet from ankles a few turns to the right and a few to the left; then up and down. Do the same with the left foot.

If your time is limited operate both feet at the same time, sitting on a chair, bed or lounge.

An elaborate explanation of the physiological effects of this exercise would take too much space and be of little service to the busy reader.

I can earnestly recommend it for cold feet, stiff ankles and toe joints, headaches resulting from various causes, catarrhal inflammation of the mucous membrane of the nostrils, etc. Provided you don't wear tight shoes this exercise V and VI can be practiced at any time with good results.

For Strong Lungs and Chest
Plate VII

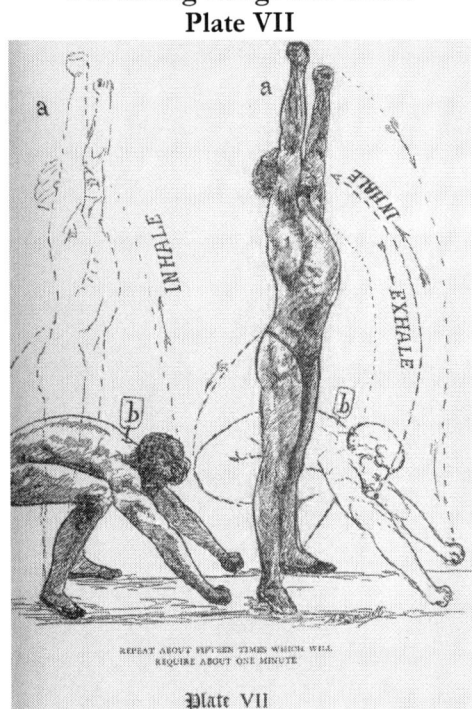

Plate VII

To cleanse the lungs of all impurities that may have accumulated during the night and increase the blood circulation:

Take two or three deep breaths, entirely emptying lungs, and then filling them to their fullest capacity. Standing erect, reach upward keeping elbows and knees straight, fists clinched or fingers outstretched as you please, and feet comfortably apart, say about the width of your shoulders. Bring the body from position A to position B repeatedly in a rather slow rhythm.

Lift chin up when in erect position A (avoid leaning backward), inhale slowly through the nose until the lungs are completely filled, elevate the shoulders as high as you can and draw the abdominal walls inward: then release abdominal walls and bring the body into position B exhaling through the nose or mouth as you please, bending the knees, bringing the armpits close to the knees or touching them if you are able to do so, attempting to touch the floor with the hands about sixteen or eighteen inches from the feet.

Abdominal Exercise
Plates VIII and IX

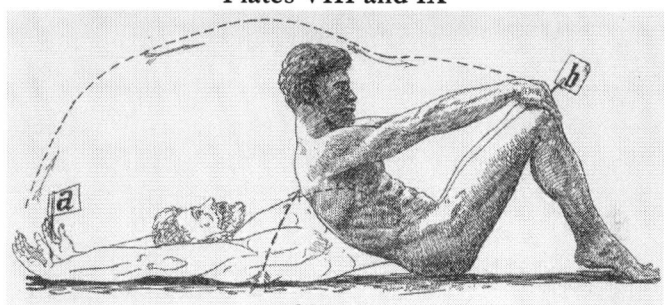

Plate VIII

To stimulate circulation in the abdominal cavity and invigorate the muscles surrounding and enfolding the assimilative and vital organs, which by reflex action of the muscles are themselves invigorated.

This exercise is practiced lying on the floor on some soft yielding but firm surface. A rug folded lengthwise or a bed-comfortable will do. An excellent exercise-mat may be made from inch or two inch pipe-felting, covered with canvas in size three by six or eight feet.

Bring the body from position A to B (or IX-C as you are able) by throwing your outstretched arms with an energetic semi-circular forward motion towards your feet or knees, following with the head and shoulders.

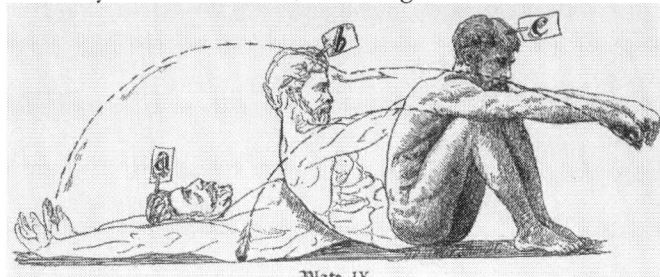

Plate IX

Avoid holding your breath while going from position A to B but expel the air from your lungs by exclaiming "whoo"; this assists, as it brings the abdominal muscles into play.

Avoid relaxing the muscles suddenly when going back into position A as the jar resulting is unpleasant and not beneficial.

It may be found difficult to follow these instructions strictly at first because of a certain amount of stiffness in the knees, hips, spine and shoulder joints, or weakness in the abdominal muscles, which are to be looked for in people of sedentary habits.

But no matter how little progress you make at first, steadily persist in your efforts to overcome these conditions and you will be amply rewarded.

Stout men will lose a great deal of superfluous fat around the waist line in attempting this exercise, as the increase of strength of the abdominal muscles destroys all fatty tissues which hamper their action.

If you are not able to reach to your knees without lifting the feet from the ground, lift them or reach only to the thighs, but try to do better next time.

The gradual development of the abdominal muscles insures a safeguard against ruptures.

The number of consecutive exercises of this kind must depend upon the condition and good judgment of the reader. Should your limit be five, then rest a few seconds and take five more and so on until you have taken twenty-five or exercised in this way for at least two or three minutes.

I would impress upon my reader the great importance of this kind of exercise to health.

For Back Muscles and Spine
Plate X

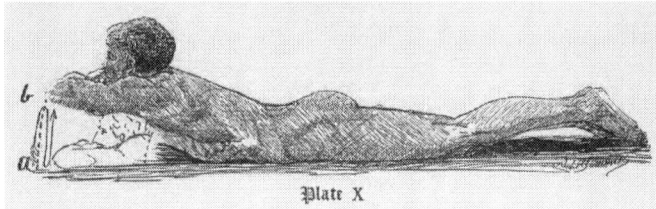

Plate X

As the reverse of exercise VIII or IX in which the abdominal muscles are chiefly involved and the spine strongly and repeatedly brought into a convex curve, take the following exercise for the back muscles and spine.

Lie on your abdomen with the legs in a comfortable position, chin (or forehead) resting on the folded arms.

Consecutively raise elbows, head and chest together (the chin or forehead not leaving the arms during the exercise) from two to nine inches, according to your ability, from A to B as shown in illustration, with a spring-like motion, not stopping at A. Avoid striking the floor with the elbows; put the energy in the rising motion. The lumbar region is thus vigorously brought into action.

Remark: Practice this exercise with forehead resting on arms, if not able to occupy illustrated position, until joints in neck gain suppleness.

Persons past middle age will probably have some difficulty in raising higher than an inch or two at first and will feel exhausted after five or six consecutive attempts. They should rest a few seconds after four or five exercises, but increase the height of the rise and the number of times in proportion with their gain of muscular strength and suppleness of spine. One minute will be sufficient.

Few minutes spent daily in this exercise will soon result in correcting the round backs which are caused by sitting with in-sunken chest, by exaggerated bicycle riding, etc.

I have given this exercise with surprising results, even to men of sixty years of age.

Natural Massage Exercise for Exhilaration
Plate XI

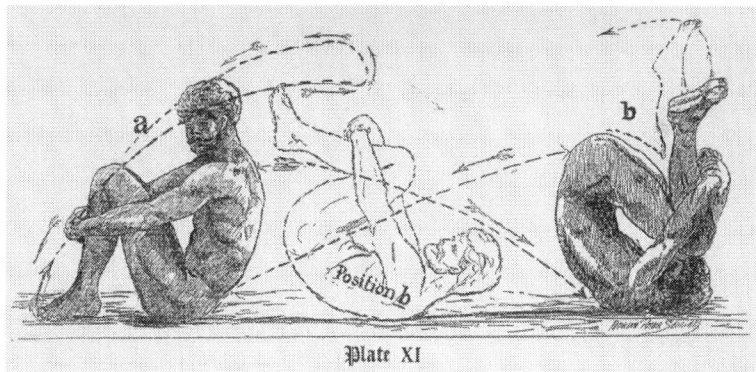

Plate XI

This exercise is rather difficult to illustrate, but simple in execution.

It is like a rocking chair in motion, the spine being the rocker. The body is doubled up as shown in illustration and this attitude is kept throughout the massage exercise.

Start this exercise by sitting down, clasping the hands below the knees, roll into position B and, without stopping there, roll back into the sitting position without unclasping your hands or changing the convex curve of your spine; in other words, throw your body from the sitting position A into shoulder position B and back into A with an uninterrupted rolling motion, occupying about three seconds. Repeat two or three minutes, taking an occasional rest so that your breathing may become normal.

Don't hold your breath, but breathe as naturally as possible.

The Bath
Plate XII

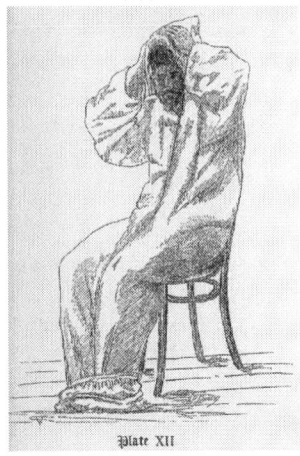

Plate XII

That the tonic effect of a cold bath upon the nervous system may be fully obtained, it should always be preceded by sufficient exercise to put the body in a glow; but do not take your bath until you breathe naturally and the heart has resumed its normal action.

It should be taken in such a manner as to wet the body all over, beginning with the head, then shoulders, chest, back and limbs, requiring in all only from two to six seconds.

Before rubbing yourself, cover every part of your body with a bath robe or bath sheet made of Turkish toweling, which is preferable to any other material because it will absorb the water rapidly. (If you have no such robe or sheet get into bed.)

Do not fail to cover your feet also, that they may feel the general reaction which follows immediately upon covering yourself with the bath robe.

Rub your hair well with a towel until dry (it strengthens the roots of the hair) and then after the reaction has fully taken place rub any part of the body that feels wet and follow this by a general friction with your hands or a towel, beginning with the limbs and following with the trunk, shoulders and arms.

I wish to emphasize the benefit derived from thoroughly wrapping up the body after the cold water application. It hastens the reaction and makes it uniform, as it checks the loss of heat all over the body at the same time. This is of special importance to people who are not in vigorous health.

Those who think that cold water baths do not agree with them will probably change their opinion after a trial of this method.

The writer hopes that he has redeemed his promise of a few simple suggestions and that their value will be appreciated by all who make use of them.

Printed in Great Britain
by Amazon